The Enlightenment Pie Food Journal

Lisa M Gunshore

BALBOA.PRESS
A DIVISION OF HAY HOUSE

Balboa Press books may be ordered through booksellers or by contacting:

Balboa Press
A Division of Hay House
1663 Liberty Drive
Bloomington, IN 47403
www.balboapress.com
844-682-1282

·Because of the dynamic nature of the Internet, any web addresses or
links contained in this book may have changed since publication and
may no longer be valid. The views expressed in this work are solely those
of the author and do not necessarily reflect the views of the publisher,
and the publisher hereby disclaims any responsibility for them.

The author of this book does not dispense medical advice or prescribe the use
of any technique as a form of treatment for physical, emotional, or medical
problems without the advice of a physician, either directly or indirectly. The
intent of the author is only to offer information of a general nature to help
you in your quest for emotional and spiritual well-being. In the event you use
any of the information in this book for yourself, which is your constitutional
right, the author and the publisher assume no responsibility for your actions.

Any people depicted in stock imagery provided by Getty Images are
models, and such images are being used for illustrative purposes only.
Certain stock imagery © Getty Images.

Print information available on the last page.

ISBN: 978-1-9822-6318-8 (sc)
ISBN: 978-1-9822-6317-1 (e)

Balboa Press rev. date: 02/15/2021

Contents

Statement of Intent

As a Holistic Health Practitioner and Medical Intuitive I present eating and healthy living options. I suggest nutritional changes based on established resources such as www.candidadiet.org and the mold diet as suggested by Dr. Schoemaker[1]. I am certified in Nutritional Cooking and hold an A.A.S. degree in Culinary Arts and consequently offer sound cooking advice and culinary nutrition information. I help clients incorporate healthy, vitamin and nutrient rich foods into meals. I will teach you, the reader, about phytonutrients and healthy fats. I am neither a medical doctor nor a registered dietician. I will not prescribe, diagnose, or cure any disease or medical issue. While I may suggest nutritional supplements to enhance your healthy lifestyle, I will not prescribe supplements to treat a medical condition. It is very important to have your own team of doctors to support any medical diagnosis or treatment. My counseling and intuitive guidance is meant to support your current medical advice and to enhance your healthy lifestyle overall. This book is intended to be a resource and is not meant to re-create any diet or to offer medical advice. This book shares the knowledge I have gained through research I have done in regard to mold and candida diets, supplementation, and food.

---

[1] Ritchie Shoemaker, M. D., is a recognized leader in patient care, research and education pioneer in the field of biotoxin related illness. http://www.survivingmold.com/about/ritchie-shoemaker-m-d

Statement of Belief

I am a fourth generation psychic medium. I was raised Irish Catholic and confirmed in the Catholic Church. In 2010 I converted to Vajrayana Buddhism. It is my belief that God and all Sentient Beings are interconnected. I believe there is a world beyond time and space we may never fully understand as Human Beings, yet we are able to tap into this world through our conscious and unconscious minds. Learning about religion, belief, psychic phenomena, and so on, is ongoing and there is always more to understand. Although I am a Psychic and I understand the many facets of the Occult; I do not identify with Paganism, Wicca or other Occult religions. I currently practice Vajrayana Buddhism, and the Middle Way is what I try to incorporate in my daily life. I have an appreciation for my Catholic upbringing and the family values I learned growing up. I respect all religions as they have something to offer the open mind. My belief is that all things are an interconnected web of Divine energy.

Reader Intention

For those who are searching for Truth beyond the mundane, beyond Samsara[2].

For those who have run out of hope and are searching for the light.

For those who are hungry for knowledge, wisdom and truth.

For those whose souls have committed to a greater calling.

For those who wish to serve the greater good and humanity.

For the warriors[3] who are willing to confront their obstacles and fears head on.

For those who have lost trust in the system and are looking for inner peace, depth, knowledge and understanding.

And So It Is.

---

[2] Samsara is the cycle of death and rebirth to which life in the material world is bound.

[3] Warrior here is defined by *Shambhala: The Sacred Path of the Warrior* written by Chogyam Trunpa Rinpoche. To purchase https://www.amazon.com/dp/B00HEN3JHW/ref=dp-kindle-redirect?_encoding=UTF8&btkr=1

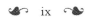

Objective

Living in Vitality

It seems everywhere we look these days; we see more and more people carrying weight. To someone on the outside they may only see the unhealthy side effects of poor diet and pass judgements on the person's ability to care for themselves. What may not be seen is the deep layers of emotional baggage that this person is carrying and their lack of Self Love that ultimately affects their choices when caring or ultimately 'not caring' for themselves. The baggage is really layering that we have acquired throughout this lifetime and others and it has manifested into; physical weight that we carry in our bodies, emotional weight, and spiritual weight in the form of karma.

The Enlightenment Pie Food journal has been created to serve as a workbook in conjunction with Enlightenment Pie. This journal represents step one of the Enlightenment Pie process; become aware. To become aware is to practice mindfulness, learn how to be mindful of both your physical body and your emotional body in relation to your food choices and your weight, and to learn basic meditation and contemplative practices to help you move through your inner work with ease and apply your learnings in your daily life.

This journal gives you space to write down your thoughts

that come from the self-inquiry questions and contemplative practices throughout the book. Included are short recaps of the activities from Enlightenment Pie to help guide you through the journal and answer the tough questions throughout. At the back of the journal you have thirty food sensitivity tracking templates. This allows you to track how your food and your emotions are impacting you throughout a thirty-day time period.

Enlightenment Pie is a process to teach you how to release weight from your Spirit, mind and body. I have learned from my own experience that to truly 'lose weight' we must complete the inner work in ALL aspects of our lives. By looking at those difficult pieces of ourselves that is our weight; we bring to the surface many destructive emotions. By working through these emotions and facing them - rather than 'stuffing them away'; we are able to overcome this weight once and for all. This journal is not really about changing your diet but instead transforming all aspects of your Self and changing your life!

In this journal I outline the process of completing inner work to heal the baggage that is affecting your weight:

1. Meditation – Learn the basics of meditation to help you move through your inner work with ease and how to incorporate practice into your daily life. Practice mindfulness. Learn how to be mindful of both your physical body and your emotional body in relation to your food choices and your weight. Begin to build a relationship with your physical body and be able to listen and understand its needs.
2. Journaling – Learn how to utilize journaling and self-inquiry to come to the root block of your body and yourself. Practice self-inquiry through the exercises in the journal.
3. Food Sensitivity Tracking Template - Learn how to begin the process of managing your food allergies and how your emotional state can affect your food choices.

Building Your Spiritual Foundation

WHEN YOU BEGIN TO MAKE a crust you first cut sticks of butter into flour. You can do this with a fork, with a pastry cutter, or your fingers. The goal is to create small pea sized balls of flour and butter. You then add milk or water until it becomes a dough. You are taking three forms; liquid, fat and wheat, and making it into one form that is stronger and able to withstand the baking process while holding in a filling. It is important not to overwork the dough or it will become stiff and will not be the flaky crust you want; but instead become hard and chewy. Although there are only 3 ingredients in a pie crust, it can be very easy to ruin it; by adding too much of one ingredient or by mixing too much or too little.

The process of making pie crust can be likened to the process of bringing your health into balance. You begin with simple ingredients that together can build a spiritual foundation. This journal encompasses the ingredients of Step One of the Enlightenment Pie process; Become Aware. Awareness rises from spiritual practices that bring you into the present moment. This journal is your crust. If you overwork yourself in this process your energy will become static and the work will become hard. Giving just the right amount of time and energy into building your foundation will bring about the desired result.

**To achieve perfect health; you must be balanced.
To be balanced; you must build a foundation
of practice that develops awareness.
As you begin those practices; you
must still create balance.**

The tools given here are providing you with behaviors that you will carry for a lifetime. They are the tools that you will go back to again and again. In the hardest of times it is the simplest of practices that can have the most profound effect. By mixing these tools together, you are creating a foundation to 'hold' all the pieces or 'filling' in your life together.

Just like there are ingredients in a pie crust; there are tools that provide the foundation for healing. A tool belt to create awareness. This is the natural place to begin as the journey to awareness unfolds through this process. Whatever you are going through in your life whether it be physical, spiritual, mental or emotional; these behaviors are what will act as a guide to release you from your suffering. Once you learn and understand how to put these practices into place you will find that they can move you through a crisis with ease and will provide some comfort in times that are uncomfortable.

The five practices for your spiritual foundation are:

1. Creating Sacred Space
2. Meditation
3. Contemplation
4. Journaling
5. Self-Inquiry

Create Sacred Space

"This is my simple religion. There is no need for temples, no need for complicated philosophies. Our brain, our own heart is our temple; the philosophy is kindness." HH Dalai Lama

A SACRED SPACE IS DEFINED AS a space distinguished from all other spaces. A space where all the actions, thoughts and intentions within this space can bear spiritual meaning. Sacred space is where you can meditate, journal, throw an oracle card or even just sit in contemplation. It is a space that you journey to when you need to think, when you need to cry, or when you need to light a candle for a friend in need. By returning to the same location time and again you create a vibration, or an energy in that space. This is an energy of healing and of light; of intuitiveness and of creativity. Just like a writer may have a writing room or a painter a studio; you too want to have sacred space. And you can have more than one. You can have a favorite garden outside and a favorite chair inside. You can go all out and have an altar with candles and deities and cards and incense, or simply light a candle in your bedroom. The beauty of your sacred space is that it is just that; your own.

As I was writing about sacred space I went for a walk on my usual trail by the creek. I always walk 3 miles out and then loop back. At the three-mile point there is a dirt path that connects to the sidewalk. It leads down a small hill to a sandy bank on the side of the creek. I love this space. I sit and meditate and have, at times, even done yoga creek side. There are many tall trees. The creek is wide in this particular location and breaks in the middle where a tall tree has grown right out of the water. Last spring there was a Beaver damn here and I even had the blessing of seeing the Beavers before they tore it down and moved on. On this particular day it felt much like fall. The sun was shining, and it was warm. However, the air was crisp and smelled of burnt wood. The leaves on the trees had changed to golds and even browns and some of them were even scattered on the ground. I sat down next to my favorite tree with my feet dangling above the water. There was a slight breeze. You could hear the rustling of the leaves and the water flowing and bubbling around itself and the big tree in the center of the creek. At that moment I thought to myself how wonderful this space was. How blessed I was to be sitting there at that moment. It was not long before that moment that I was feeling completely out of sorts. Now here I was feeling healthy and had found some peace. I took in the scene with a deep breath and instead of closing my eyes to meditate I just watched. I watched a golden leaf spiral in the currents of the water as it floated past me. I watched the birds fly back and forth between the almost barren trees. I saw the sunlight shown through the trees and sparkle on the water's edge. I listened also. I listened to the sound of the wind. It told me that winter was coming, and this moment would soon be gone. The energy of that moment and that space felt like home to me. It felt warm and soft and comforting. This space had become very dear to me over the year that I have lived there, and many tears, joys and healings had taken place there.

This is a perfect example of sacred space. It does not have to be an altar that you create or barrier in your home just for meditating. It is a special place. A place where you feel at home. A place where you can take your troubles and your joys and 'hold' them there until you are ready to release them. It can be likened to a mothers' womb where everything is sacred and life-giving...a creative force that no one can name or point out but instead you must sense it. It is filled with the energy of the heart. Opening the center of all seven centers filling you with healing, compassion and light.

It is not necessary to create Sacred Space; you carry it within you.

It may reveal itself in nature, in a statue of a Goddess, in a favorite chair or in a scent you cannot forget. Sacred Space is that place where you feel one with God and ultimately connected to yourself.

Where or What is my Sacred Space?

_____

_____

_____

_____

_____

_____

_____

_____

_____

_____

_____

_____

_____

_____

_____

_____

_____

_____

_____

_____

_____

_____

_____

_____

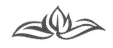

Meditation

"Why are we so petrified of silence? Here, can you handle this?...Did you think about your bills, your ex, your deadlines; or when you think you're gonna die. Or did you long for the next distraction?" Alanis Morrisette

M EDITATION IS THE ACT OF coming in to the present moment through breath and focused intention. Meditation is where we connect to our Truth. Truth with a capital T is defined by one of the Yamas in the Yoga Sutra, Satya. Satya encourages us to live and speak our truth at all times. This idea of truth is about understanding the difference between making a judgment through one's own perception and actual observation of reality or the facts of a situation through growing self-awareness. Meditation brings self-awareness by coming into a present state called mindfulness. Mindfulness is focused awareness in the present moment in order to accept your feelings, thoughts and sensations in a calm state. Meditation and mindfulness practice are the actions that lead to consciousness.

The practice of meditation can take a lifetime of practice and still not be perfected. And perfection should not be the goal. Instead strive to connect with your Self, become neutral and listen to your inner voice. Remove the notion that the mind will be totally clear after a few deep breaths. Meditation is less about clearing the mind and instead, watching the mind. You may find that when you first clear your mind then the inner world begins to speak, filling you with all sorts of new pictures and ideas, your shopping list or anything else your mind wants reviewing. Are you staring into a blank space? No, of course not. You are just listening and becoming aware of what is there deep inside you vs. the chatter from the outside world.

Meditation practice begins with breathing exercises. The first thing that may come to mind when you think of meditation is a picture of a person sitting in lotus position with their eyes closed and their mind clear. There is no need for this. Sit in a comfortable chair, lie on the floor…the only thing I don't recommend is lying in bed. You are sure to fall asleep! Now, if you do fall asleep when trying to meditate; give yourself permission! You are obviously tired. I once had a student that fell asleep every time she meditated for the first 3 months! She finally caught up on the rest her body needed from years of working long hours and was able to hold a concentrated meditation. Whatever you do, as you go through the process; do NOT beat yourself up for doing something 'wrong'. The beauty of this work is that nothing is 'wrong'. Everything happens exactly as it should. Being aware of your experience is the process.

Once you are comfortably situated begin to breathe. Just begin by breathing normally. Notice your belly. When you breathe in, your belly should fill with air. When you breathe out, it should go in. Most Americans breathe incorrectly. You may find right away that you are not filling up the lungs and diaphragm area properly. A great technique is to lay flat on a flat surface; such as the floor or even a table. Breathe in and out. Feel your stomach. Where is the air going? How does it feel? How deep does the breath go? Ideally you want to fill up the diaphragm in the lower abdomen first, then the lungs, and then as your release; you release the lungs first, then the diaphragm. It takes practice just to breathe. You would be surprised at how much work that can take. The diaphragm is a muscle just like any other and you will need to 'work it out' for a while before you feel you can take deep breaths. I read a statistic once that we only have about 40% fresh air in our lungs at a time. If you can get yourself to a point where you breathe in for 8 counts, out for 8 counts, 8 times in a row; you will then 100% fresh air in your lungs. You may also be dizzy, but it is great for refreshing the lungs and releasing toxins.

A great breathing technique is 'in and out' breathing. It is the process of breathing in through the nose and out through the mouth. The purpose of this is that the nose provides a natural filter so the air you are bringing in is more concentrated and is cleaner. When you release from the mouth you are truly releasing and relaxing the body. Spend some quality time with your breath. Notice how your lungs and diaphragm feel and notice how clear your mind is when you are thinking so hard about breathing and nothing else.

Once you have practiced your breathing technique; the next piece of meditation is clearing the mind in order to come into the present moment. First go back to your breathing to begin the process of clearing the mind and body. The next practice you can add to this is mindfulness of the physical body. Notice your body. Have you ever had a bruise just show up and you don't remember how it got there? Being aware of your physical body can be a real eye opener. Notice where you hurt or have aches. Notice where you feel good. Notice how you are sitting or lying down. Just notice. You can also do this with your emotional and energy bodies. How do you feel? How does your energy feel? You do not need to know anything about energy to do this exercise. You inherently 'know' what is energetically blocked or stuck in your field. Just ask yourself and it will come to you. Mindfulness and breathing are two great ways to get started with your meditation. It will automatically clear a lot of thoughts that were running through your mind before you sat down.

The next thing that you can do is begin to notice your thoughts. You might be thinking - I hope I can get my mind clear while I try this meditation thing. Or, I hope my dog doesn't start barking while I am trying to be quiet. Recognize the thought and watch it as though it did not belong to you. A favorite visualization technique to clear the mind I recommend using is the balloon technique. Imagine the thought in a balloon. Then float it away. This sends the energy and the thought away bringing your mind back to the present. You can also flush these thoughts down the toilet or various other visualization techniques you may wish to use. The idea is to clear it from your mind, so you come back to the present moment.

Becoming mindful of your body in the present moment and clearing your thoughts are the basics of beginning meditation. Utilize the practice of meditation when you are completing mindfulness practices or working on self-inquiry questions. Meditation will help you become centered and your responses to the questions will be more neutral and less from an egoic state.

Practice Meditation and Belly Breathing each day for seven days; 15 minutes or more a day.

What do you notice about meditation? Write down your thoughts, challenges and changes over the seven days.

_____

_____

_____

_____

_____

_____

_____

_____

_____

_____

_____

_____

_____

_____

_____

_____

_____

_____

_____

_____

_____

_____

_____

_____

_____

_____

_____

_____

_____

Contemplation

"What we plant in the soil of contemplation, we shall reap in the harvest of action." Meister Eckhart

WHENEVER I HEAR THE WORD contemplation; I think of the Monty Python skit where philosophers are playing soccer. As soon as the whistle blows; instead of playing they all put their hands to their chin and begin contemplating. Finally, one of them gets an idea and kicks the ball and scores. While this is a comedy skit, it accurately portrays the practice of contemplation. Rather than 'reacting' to a situation in your life, you think about it instead. Contemplation is the choice to take the time to 'hold' a situation or an idea in your mind before you take action. This not only prevents you from doing something stupid but can also provide you with an answer or a solution totally different than what you expected. It is really a process of slowing down and taking stock rather than acting rashly or from an emotional space. How many times have you done something out of fear, worry or stress; rather than out of a peaceful state of the heart? How many times have you gone to bed and awoke in the morning realizing that you would have done something totally different than you did the night before?

I'd like to use a pie analogy to further explain contemplation. If you make a pie and serve it before it's cooked…it is just not going to be good. You put a pie in the oven, and it bakes. The oven 'holds' it for an hour or so. It keeps it in a safe space where it takes everything that you put together and solidifies it. When you take it out, it has been fully cooked. You then set the pie on a rack and let it cool. Again, another resting period. Finally, it is time to cut into it and serve it. Contemplation represents that baking period. You begin with an idea or a situation; a question or an issue that needs resolution. You take it and 'hold' it. Just like the oven holds the pie. The issue will sit in your consciousness for an hour, a day or even a week or month depending on what it is. There is no need to think about it all the time or even to write about it all the time. Just by choosing to 'hold' it, you are doing just that. You may have dreams about it. You may journal about it. You may wake up one morning and know the answer. The idea behind it is that when it is 'cooked' you will become totally clear on what to do. Once you know what to do there is again a 'cooling' or resting period. You write down what it is that you are to do and leave it yet again. You allow it to manifest in the right time with right action. Then you act on the information you received. Let's say you have a fight with a friend. Our natural reaction is to try and fix it right away. Can you imagine waiting and instead contemplating your next step? Once you know what that is can you imagine waiting just a bit longer before acting on it? You will not react the way you would have in the moment and you will not solve it the way you originally intended. By waiting you also eliminated much of the drama that may have occurred had you continued to push the situation.

When you are completing self-inquiry exercises you will want to use contemplation to gather information. You ask yourself a question and then you think about it. Our first reaction to a question asked of oneself is usually reactionary and from the egoic mind. Allowing the question to simmer in your consciousness for a period of time can benefit you because you will push past your own ego and Truth will rise up revealing what is really behind these tough questions. Journaling your thoughts through the contemplative process is an important action because you will want to note all your thoughts so you can begin to identify the patterns of your egoic mind and begin to separate those from your inherent Truth.

Contemplative practice: Contemplate your current state of health and overall happiness. What conclusions do you draw from this exercise? How do you think you want things to change? What arises as you think about your happiness?

_____

_____

_____

_____

_____

_____

_____

_____

_____

_____

_____

_____

_____

Lisa M Gunshore

_____

_____

_____

_____

_____

_____

_____

_____

_____

_____

_____

_____

Journaling

D O YOU KEEP A DIARY or write in a journal? You may have two or three journals you have either bought, or been given, just lying around your house. A percentage of those journals just lying around may have writing in the first two or three pages and the rest is left blank. There are a small percentage of people who write in a journal every day and are diligent in this practice. Journaling can feel like a chore. It can be tough to create a journaling routine and carving time out for it with our busy schedules can be a challenge. Just like meditation, journaling is an important tool to generate awareness and creative flow. Morning is the best time to write. You experience more of a stream of consciousness when you first wake up. That said, how and when you journal is up to you. I have one student who has a different journal for each thing she writes; one for homework, one for dreams, one for books she is reading and so on. I have another student who has the most beautiful journals and she writes fluidly in them until they are full. Then there is me; who has notepads on her desk, journals in her bed, computers on her lap, and a small notebook in my kitchen. My husband journals on an app called Day One. It is an excellent mobile app if you are looking to switch to a digital version of journaling. I still prefer my composition notebooks and mechanical pencils, but I am working on making the technology switch.

Journaling can provide a deep connection within yourself.

Writing can also move energy. If you are sad and you write it all down, it will not only aid in clearing what triggered the emotion from your mind, but it has also been proven that it can release blocks from your energy field. If you are mad, writing it out can diffuse the anger and even provide a solution to your problem.

Steps to Journaling

1. Identify your preferred journaling device; app, notebook, diary
2. Identify your preferred space for journaling and time of day
3. Write and stick to it. Remember it takes 30 days to build a behavior so practice writing daily for 30 days and note in your journal how you feel as you begin to add this practice to your daily life.

Self-Inquiry

L EARNING TO MEDITATE, ALTHOUGH CHALLENGING for some, brings peace and tranquility in the midst of our busy lives. To practice contemplation and write in a journal brings answers we were not expecting and clarity to our current issues. On the other hand, self-inquiry can create tension, frustration, anger and static energy.

Self-Inquiry is one of the Niyamas from the Yoga Sutra; Svadhyaya. Svadhyaya means self-study. Self-inquiry is the act of studying yourself. This requires the act of asking yourself the questions necessary to work through your blocks such as; why am I so angry? The process of self-inquiry is the most challenging of any practice that generates awareness. It is certainly the most uncomfortable.

Self-Inquiry Steps

1. Identify the area in which you wish to work on yourself. Ie. Anger, relationship patterns, financial etc.
2. Ask yourself; how is this pattern/experience serving me? What is it teaching me?
3. Identify what you have learned from this experience or pattern and write down actionable steps you can take to honor what you have learned.

I WILL USE A SPECIFIC EXAMPLE. I have a temper. I used the process of self-inquiry to identify how anger was serving me. I wrote down in my journal what happened when I got angry, why I got angry and asked the question; what was anger providing for me that I could not provide for myself? The response from my ego was that anger serves no one. Anger is bad. However, after meditation and contemplation I realized that when I got angry, I pushed everyone away. Why was I doing this? Anger *was* serving me. Anger was providing a boundary for me when I could not. It was a major insight into my life patterns. I chose to honor my anger by learning how to say no and create functional boundaries in my life. Eventually my temper waned. Now when I get frustrated and notice my temper rising; I am aware, almost instantly, that I have allowed my boundaries to be overstepped and it was time to look at my commitments.

The art of self-study can help you understand the patterns in your life; why you need them and how to break the pattern. Once you are able to overcome the 'destructive emotions' that arise with self-inquiry; you will find release, acceptance and forgiveness.

Pie Chart Activity

Create a Pie Chart for your life.

Draw a circle on a piece of paper. This circle represents 100% of your time both awake and asleep. Contemplate what compartments exist in your life and how much time you are spending on each. Meditate on your life and look at it as though you were watching a movie. Take in how you have been living and the choices you have made. Do NOT go a step further until you have truly looked at the different aspects of your life from an honest perspective. If you do not complete this first step honestly and methodically, your work following this will be only touching the surface and will not serve you in reaching your Truth. Draw these compartments on the pie chart and complete the following self-inquiry questions.

Lisa M Gunshore

What are the compartments that make up your life?

_____

_____

_____

_____

_____

_____

_____

_____

_____

_____

_____

_____

_____

_____

_____

_____

_____

_____

_____

_____

_____

_____

_____

_____

_____

_____

_____

_____

_____

How much time are you spending on each one?

_____

_____

_____

_____

_____

_____

_____

_____

_____

_____

_____

_____

_____

_____

_____

_____

_____

_____

_____

_____

_____

_____

_____

_____

_____

_____

_____

Lisa M Gunshore

Are you creating a balance between these compartments?

_____

_____

_____

_____

_____

_____

_____

_____

_____

_____

_____

_____

_____

_____

_____

_____

_____

_____

_____

_____

_____

_____

_____

_____

_____

_____

_____

Where in my life, have I become imbalanced?
Just take that question in.
Contemplate.
Journal.
Meditate.

_____

_____

_____

_____

_____

_____

_____

_____

_____

_____

_____

_____

_____

_____

_____

What have I discovered about myself?

_____

_____

_____

_____

_____

_____

_____

_____

_____

_____

_____

_____

_____

_____

_____

_____

_____

_____

_____

_____

_____

_____

_____

_____

_____

_____

_____

_____

_____

_____

Lisa M Gunshore

How does this make me feel?

_____

_____

_____

_____

_____

_____

_____

_____

_____

_____

_____

_____

_____

_____

_____

_____

_____

_____

_____

_____

_____

_____

_____

_____

_____

_____

_____

_____

_____

_____

What is this teaching me?

_____

_____

_____

_____

_____

_____

_____

_____

_____

_____

_____

_____

_____

_____

_____

_____

_____

_____

_____

_____

_____

_____

_____

_____

_____

How have I learned from this?

_____

_____

_____

_____

_____

_____

_____

_____

_____

_____

_____

_____

_____

_____

_____

What am I not honoring within myself that has created this imbalance?

_____

_____

_____

_____

_____

_____

_____

_____

_____

_____

_____

_____

_____

_____

_____

_____

_____

_____

_____

_____

_____

_____

_____

_____

_____

_____

_____

_____

_____

What emotions come 'up' for me when I complete this exercise?

_____

_____

_____

_____

_____

_____

_____

_____

_____

_____

_____

_____

_____

_____

_____

_____

_____

_____

_____

_____

_____

_____

_____

_____

_____

_____

_____

What are these emotions teaching me?

_____

_____

_____

_____

_____

_____

_____

_____

_____

_____

_____

Lisa M Gunshore

What do I learn from these emotions?

_____

_____

_____

_____

_____

_____

_____

_____

_____

_____

_____

_____

_____

_____

_____

_____

_____

_____

_____

_____

_____

_____

_____

_____

_____

_____

_____

_____

_____

Mindfulness of the Body Activity

OUR WEIGHT LOSS JOURNEY IS a partnership between our physical body and our awareness. In the world we know today our physical bodies take a beating. We work tireless hours and are often running from place to place. We do not give ourselves time to eat or exercise properly. We find ourselves tired, overworked and often with little to no energy to maintain even the simplest health routine. In addition, we do not pay much attention to our bodies. We are not aware of what is happening to them in the present moment; our minds are always focused elsewhere.

How many times have you found a bruise or cut on your body and you do not even remember how it got there? Has your body become stiff or sore and yet you are unsure of what might have caused it? Do you sometimes feel bloated or nauseous and thought perhaps you just weren't feeling well? Do you take aspirin for a headache without wondering why the headache was there in the first place?

Getting connected with your body is a first step in discovering the cause of your weight gain and becoming acquainted with your symptoms. If aren't aware of what your body needs or how it feels; how then, can you possibly support it?

Activity

1. Sit in a chair or on a meditation cushion. Ensure your space is quiet and you will not be disturbed. Begin breathing in through your nose and out through your mouth. With each breath, breathe more deeply, taking in more and more fresh air and releasing the stale air in your lungs.
2. Place your hands on the areas of your body you are unhappy with. This could be a place where you carry weight or a place where you are experiencing pain, discomfort or dis-ease.
3. Take a deep breath and with your hands still on your body; answer the following questions.

What is my level of awareness currently? Around my health? Around my overall happiness?

_____

_____

_____

_____

_____

_____

_____

_____

_____

_____

_____

_____

_____

_____

_____

_____

_____

_____

_____

_____

_____

_____

_____

_____

_____

_____

_____

What am I using to medicate myself? Tylenol, Caffeine, Television,
Anti-depressants etc.

_____

_____

_____

_____

_____

_____

_____

_____

_____

_____

_____

_____

_____

_____

_____

_____

_____

_____

_____

_____

_____

_____

_____

_____

_____

_____

_____

_____

_____

_____

Where am I self-medicating? Constantly on the phone or out socially, alcohol etc.

_____

_____

_____

_____

_____

_____

_____

_____

_____

_____

_____

_____

Is my body physically healthy? Proper weight, proper diet, illness etc.

_____

_____

_____

_____

_____

_____

_____

_____

_____

_____

_____

_____

_____

_____

_____

Lisa M Gunshore

Am I happy?

_____

_____

_____

_____

_____

_____

_____

_____

_____

_____

_____

_____

_____

_____

_____

Lisa M Gunshore

How does my body feel?

_____

_____

_____

_____

_____

_____

_____

_____

_____

_____

_____

_____

_____

_____

Where do I feel pain? Soreness? Inflexible? Heavy?

_____

_____

_____

_____

_____

_____

_____

_____

_____

_____

_____

_____

_____

_____

_____

_____

_____

_____

_____

_____

_____

_____

_____

_____

_____

_____

_____

Where do I feel light? Open? Strong?

_____

_____

_____

_____

_____

_____

_____

_____

_____

_____

_____

_____

_____

_____

_____

_____

_____

_____

_____

_____

_____

_____

_____

_____

_____

_____

What emotion is here?

_____

_____

_____

_____

_____

_____

_____

_____

_____

_____

_____

_____

_____

_____

_____

_____

_____

_____

_____

_____

_____

_____

_____

_____

_____

_____

_____

What other messages/images/thoughts/feelings come up for me when I touch this area? For example; you may place your hands on your stomach and see a yellow light or feel the anxiety of your life being carried in this space. By becoming aware of what is going on within your own physical body, you will begin to build a relationship with it. You will begin to understand what is causing the excess weight and also what emotional issues you may need to work on. Spend at least 20-45 minutes a day with this exercise for at least 7 days. Journal what comes to you as messages/thoughts/feelings daily.

Mindfulness of the Emotional Body Activity

There is a partnership that exists between our weight on our physical body and the weight we carry in our emotional body. The emotional body is a subtle energy field that surrounds your physical body. It is also directly connected to our energy centers or chakras, as well as the other energetic bodies in our field such as our aura and our energy channels. The emotional body carries the emotion and/or baggage that we have carried in this lifetime and potentially other lifetimes as well.

Practice to examine the emotional body

Sit in a chair or on a meditation cushion. Ensure you are in a quiet space without distraction. Take a few minutes to breathe deeply, eyes closed, and place yourself in a meditative state. Once you have quieted your mind; imagine that you are made of glass. Visualize your body as though it were crystal. The idea here is that you are able to see through yourself as though it were a clear glass. Once you have that image in your mind; imagine that you are able to see your emotions on and in this crystal image. A couple of examples could be that there is a great deal of red paint on your heart, indicating that you have anger in your heart center. You could also see cracks in your glass around your throat, indicating that you have had communication issues. These are just a couple examples of the thousands of visualizations you can have on your body of glass. Take time to look at your body of glass and to take note of what you see. You may not understand what it all means at first but as information unfolds you will discover more about your emotional body and where your emotions may be sitting in your physical body.

Our emotions are a trigger when it comes to when and what we eat. Most of us have diets that are stress based. When we are stressed, frustrated, hormonal etc.; we find ourselves eating sugary foods or drinking alcohol. Self-inquiry and meditation can help you gain awareness of these triggers and begin tracking how you are emotionally eating and also getting to the deeper issues.

Homework:

Meditate on your body of glass and to begin to understand the emotions that you carry in your physical body. Utilize the following self-inquiry questions throughout the week to begin to identify your emotional contributors to your weight.

What emotions were I experiencing over this week that caused me to eat?

_____

_____

_____

_____

_____

_____

_____

_____

_____

_____

_____

_____

_____

_____

_____

_____

Lisa M Gunshore

_____

_____

_____

_____

_____

_____

_____

_____

_____

_____

_____

What did I choose to eat due to this emotion?

_____

_____

_____

_____

_____

_____

_____

_____

_____

_____

_____

_____

_____

_____

_____

_____

_____

_____

Lisa M Gunshore

_____

_____

_____

_____

_____

_____

_____

_____

_____

_____

What part of my body 'lights up' when I am eating this food?

_____

_____

_____

_____

_____

_____

_____

_____

_____

_____

_____

_____

_____

_____

_____

_____

_____

Lisa M Gunshore

_____

_____

_____

_____

_____

_____

_____

_____

_____

_____

_____

What emotion do I feel once I ate the food?

_____

_____

_____

_____

_____

_____

_____

_____

_____

_____

_____

_____

_____

_____

_____

_____

_____

Lisa M Gunshore

_____

_____

_____

_____

_____

_____

_____

_____

_____

Where does this emotion come from?

_____

_____

_____

_____

_____

_____

_____

_____

_____

_____

_____

_____

_____

_____

_____

_____

Lisa M Gunshore

How is this emotion serving me right now?

_____

_____

_____

_____

_____

_____

_____

_____

_____

_____

_____

_____

_____

_____

_____

_____

_____

Lisa M Gunshore

_____

_____

_____

_____

_____

_____

_____

_____

_____

_____

How was this process for you?

_____

_____

_____

_____

_____

_____

_____

_____

_____

_____

_____

_____

_____

_____

_____

_____

_____

_____

_____

Lisa M Gunshore

_____

_____

_____

_____

_____

_____

_____

_____

_____

_____

_____

Self-Inquiry Questions Continued

Why can't I stop myself from eating?

_____

_____

_____

_____

_____

_____

_____

_____

_____

_____

_____

_____

_____

_____

_____

Lisa M Gunshore

_____

_____

_____

_____

_____

_____

_____

_____

_____

_____

_____

Why am I unable to stop myself from eating foods I know are not good for me?

_____

_____

_____

_____

_____

_____

_____

_____

_____

_____

_____

_____

_____

_____

_____

_____

_____

Lisa M Gunshore

_____

_____

_____

_____

_____

_____

_____

_____

_____

_____

Why am I so angry?

_____

_____

_____

_____

_____

_____

_____

_____

_____

_____

_____

_____

_____

_____

_____

_____

Lisa M Gunshore

_____

_____

_____

_____

_____

_____

_____

_____

_____

_____

Where is this sadness coming from?

_____

_____

_____

_____

_____

_____

_____

_____

_____

_____

_____

_____

_____

_____

_____

_____

Lisa M Gunshore

_____

_____

_____

_____

_____

_____

_____

_____

_____

_____

Healing Your Lineage Activity

Whether we like it or not; we are our family. We carry their bloodline and more, so we carry the many genetic traits the line has within it. Our level of intelligence, our ability to connect with others, our creativity, our eating habits, our emotions; these are all pieces of the ancestral 'pie'. A student said to me, "I'm afraid if I start digging into my family history; I will not be able to come out of it and move forward." I think this is a fear in all of us. If we open up Pandora's box, will we be able to liberate ourselves from it? Or will we get stuck in the muck that it has created and be unable to achieve our authentic selves? There is no way around it. We must dig into what created us. Our family, how we were raised, and who was around us as children, are what molds us. The energy of our family shapes us into young adults. Our lineage, our bloodline, provides the framework of who we are. To liken it to a pie; our lineage is the flour in the makings of the crust and our experiences with our family in this life as young children, is the butter that holds the flour in place.

Begin to investigate your ancestry by evaluating your childhood and coming to an understanding of your relationship with your family in the present. Your relationship with your parents or caregivers is a starting point. Who influenced you the most? How have your parents and/or caregivers impacted you and your life? If you were to look back at your early years of childhood, from as early as you remember to about 12; who were you closest with? Do you remember the first time you felt resentment towards your parents? Do you remember the time they were most proud? When did you feel understood by your parents? Have you ever felt understood?

Lisa M Gunshore

Activity

From a seated position, go into meditation. Then reach into the filing cabinets of your memory and pull out the last time you saw your parents. You can focus this exercise on your mother or your father or both, whichever feels right to you. You can also focus your energy on a step-parent, teacher or caregiver instead or in addition. Journal what comes up for you when you begin this meditation and answer the following self-inquiry questions.

What was it like the last time you saw them?

_____

_____

_____

_____

_____

_____

_____

_____

_____

_____

_____

_____

_____

_____

_____

_____

Lisa M Gunshore

_____

_____

_____

_____

_____

_____

_____

_____

_____

_____

How did you feel? What was the energy?

_____

_____

_____

_____

_____

_____

_____

_____

_____

_____

_____

_____

_____

_____

_____

_____

_____

_____

Lisa M Gunshore

_____

_____

_____

_____

_____

_____

_____

_____

_____

_____

_____

What was the conversation like?

_____

_____

_____

_____

_____

_____

_____

_____

_____

_____

_____

_____

_____

_____

_____

_____

_____

_____

Lisa M Gunshore

Then dig into the filing cabinet again and look at the first time you remember feeling resentment towards your parent(s). What happened?

_____

_____

_____

_____

_____

_____

_____

_____

_____

_____

_____

_____

_____

_____

_____

_____

_____

Lisa M Gunshore

_____

_____

_____

_____

_____

_____

_____

_____

_____

_____

_____

What do you remember about that time? How did you feel? How did they react?

_____

_____

_____

_____

_____

_____

_____

_____

_____

_____

_____

_____

_____

_____

_____

_____

_____

Lisa M Gunshore

_____

_____

_____

_____

_____

_____

_____

_____

_____

_____

Then take yourself back to a time you remember your parent(s) feeling proud of you? What was the achievement? How did they make you feel?

_____

_____

_____

_____

_____

_____

_____

_____

_____

_____

_____

_____

_____

_____

_____

_____

Lisa M Gunshore

_____

_____

_____

_____

_____

_____

_____

_____

_____

_____

_____

Go back further yet into your memory file to the time when you were an infant. Although you may not remember specifics; how did you feel as a baby? What was your relationship with your parents? What is your sense about that time? Were you happy? Were your parents happy?

_____

_____

_____

_____

_____

_____

_____

_____

_____

_____

_____

_____

_____

_____

_____

_____

Lisa M Gunshore

Lastly, take yourself back into the womb. What was it like to be in your mother's belly? How did you feel? How did your mother feel? Take some deep cleansing breaths and journal your experience.

_____

_____

_____

_____

_____

_____

_____

_____

_____

_____

_____

_____

_____

_____

_____

_____

_____

Lisa M Gunshore

_____

_____

_____

_____

_____

_____

_____

_____

_____

_____

_____

Activity

Write down the names of your ancestors and their date of birth going back seven generations. You can do only the female side or only the male side or both depending on what you feel you need to work on. Meditate on those names. You can even light a candle and ask those ancestors to come in to your space. If you have pictures of them put them up as a mandala to meditate on them. Place your left palm on Mother Earth. Invite your spirit guide, ancestor teachers and/or Spirit into the right palm facing upwards. Ask to please remove the genes from the ancestor that are blocking you or affecting you adversely and feel them release into the Earth. Notice what you feel and note them here.

_____

_____

_____

_____

_____

_____

_____

_____

_____

_____

Lisa M Gunshore

Create a prayer or affirmation around your lineage. What do you want to heal? What do you want to know?

Lisa M Gunshore

_____

_____

_____

_____

_____

_____

_____

_____

_____

_____

_____

Continued Self-Inquiry Questions

What is it I am really craving?

_____

_____

_____

_____

_____

_____

_____

_____

_____

_____

_____

_____

_____

_____

_____

_____

Lisa M Gunshore

_____

_____

_____

_____

_____

_____

_____

_____

_____

_____

Why am I not satisfied?

_____

_____

_____

_____

_____

_____

_____

_____

_____

_____

_____

_____

_____

_____

_____

_____

_____

_____

Lisa M Gunshore

_____

_____

_____

_____

_____

_____

_____

_____

_____

_____

What is this experience teaching me?

_____

_____

_____

_____

_____

_____

_____

_____

_____

_____

_____

_____

_____

_____

_____

_____

_____

Lisa M Gunshore

Am I lonely?

_____

_____

_____

_____

_____

_____

_____

_____

_____

_____

_____

_____

_____

_____

_____

_____

_____

_____

Lisa M Gunshore

_____

_____

_____

_____

_____

_____

_____

_____

_____

_____

How am I feeding my loneliness?

_____

_____

_____

_____

_____

_____

_____

_____

_____

_____

_____

_____

_____

_____

_____

Lisa M Gunshore

_____

_____

_____

_____

_____

_____

_____

_____

_____

When was the last time I felt really good? Physically? Emotionally? Mentally?

_____

_____

_____

_____

_____

_____

_____

_____

_____

_____

_____

_____

_____

_____

_____

_____

Lisa M Gunshore

When was the last time I felt strong?

_____

_____

_____

_____

_____

_____

_____

_____

_____

_____

_____

_____

_____

_____

_____

_____

Lisa M Gunshore

_____

_____

_____

_____

_____

_____

_____

_____

_____

_____

How often do I have the energy to exercise within my day? Even when I have to work?

_____

_____

_____

_____

_____

_____

_____

_____

_____

_____

_____

_____

_____

_____

_____

_____

_____

Lisa M Gunshore

How often do I feel really good even after eating a meal?

Lisa M Gunshore

How often have I been sick with something in the last year? Cold etc.

_____

_____

_____

_____

_____

_____

_____

_____

_____

_____

_____

_____

_____

_____

_____

_____

_____

Lisa M Gunshore

_____

_____

_____

_____

_____

_____

_____

_____

_____

_____

What tempts me?

_____

_____

_____

_____

_____

_____

_____

_____

_____

_____

_____

_____

_____

_____

_____

_____

_____

_____

Lisa M Gunshore

_____

_____

_____

_____

_____

_____

_____

_____

_____

Have I forgiven myself?

_____

_____

_____

_____

_____

_____

_____

_____

_____

_____

_____

_____

_____

_____

_____

_____

_____

_____

Lisa M Gunshore

_____

_____

_____

_____

_____

_____

_____

_____

_____

_____

Have I risked my Self? Why?

_____

_____

_____

_____

_____

_____

_____

_____

_____

_____

_____

_____

_____

_____

_____

_____

Lisa M Gunshore

_____

_____

_____

_____

_____

_____

_____

_____

_____

List your labels, traits, personalities etc. What are they doing for you? How are they serving you?

_____

_____

_____

_____

_____

_____

_____

_____

_____

_____

_____

_____

_____

_____

_____

_____

Lisa M Gunshore

_____

_____

_____

_____

_____

_____

_____

_____

_____

_____

_____

What do you learn from this?

_____

_____

_____

_____

_____

_____

_____

_____

_____

_____

_____

_____

_____

_____

_____

_____

Lisa M Gunshore

_____

_____

_____

_____

_____

_____

_____

_____

_____

_____

What image do you reflect? Is what you see when you look out the same as when others look in? Who are we projecting?

Lisa M Gunshore

_____

_____

_____

_____

_____

_____

_____

_____

_____

Food Allergies

It is very important to begin to understand what foods are serving you and what foods are not. Most of us have food sensitivities and/or food allergies. There are foods that make our bodies bloat, foods that cause diarrhea and some foods that also make us feel strong or give us extra energy. It is important to begin to build a relationship with your food. By knowing what works for your body and what doesn't; you will begin to understand how to 'feed' your body properly and will eliminate the constant up and down cycle created by eating food that creates negative vibrations in your system.

Utilize the Food Sensitivity Tracking Templates at the back of this journal to track your eating habits and emotional triggers for thirty days. This will support you in tracking what and when you are eating to better understand how food affects you physically and emotionally. Begin to notice patterns of behavior; i.e. I was stressed so I ate a cookie, or I feel bloated each time I eat cheese. Through food journaling you will begin to see how to change your diet to nurture your body vs. punish it.

There are many belief systems around nutrition and diet. Regardless of diet theories, it is important to begin to eliminate those foods that make you feel unwell. There is a significant amount of people in the United States who have become Gluten and Dairy intolerant. When working with individual clients I recommend eliminating these items from your diet completely in addition to allergy testing and supplement regimes.

If you can afford the testing for food allergies, I highly recommend it. Obtaining accurate data about your body is the most precise. However, if you keep a proper food journal you can save on testing and keep to a budget. My recommendation is to have the blood work done through a Functional Medicine doctor or nutritionist.

Spend time throughout the thirty days watching your

behaviors and becoming aware of your physical body and its needs. You will gain a much better perspective on what has been working for you and what you need to change. The goal here is to come into relationship with your body and your food. This relationship will empower you to nourish yourself. Complete the following self-inquiry questions as you come to the end of your thirty-day tracking period.

How do I feel about my progress over the past few weeks?

_____

_____

_____

_____

_____

_____

_____

_____

_____

_____

_____

_____

_____

_____

_____

_____

Lisa M Gunshore

_____

_____

_____

_____

_____

_____

_____

_____

_____

_____

What goals have I accomplished? Where am I still stuck?

_____

_____

_____

_____

_____

_____

_____

_____

_____

_____

_____

_____

_____

_____

_____

_____

Lisa M Gunshore

_____

_____

_____

_____

_____

_____

_____

_____

_____

_____

_____

What would I like to see transform over the next 8 weeks as I continue to put these tools into practice?

_____

_____

_____

_____

_____

_____

_____

_____

_____

_____

_____

_____

_____

Lisa M Gunshore

Where do I feel I still need support?

_____

_____

_____

_____

_____

_____

_____

_____

_____

_____

_____

_____

_____

_____

_____

_____

_____

Lisa M Gunshore

What can I learn about myself from this?

_____

_____

_____

_____

_____

_____

_____

_____

_____

_____

_____

_____

_____

_____

_____

_____

_____

_____

Lisa M Gunshore

_____

_____

_____

_____

_____

_____

_____

_____

_____

_____

What has been my 'aha' moment around my 'weight'?

_____

_____

_____

_____

_____

_____

_____

_____

_____

_____

_____

_____

_____

_____

Lisa M Gunshore

_____

_____

_____

_____

_____

_____

_____

_____

_____

_____

Conclusion

I have given you some basic tools to use in your daily life and have offered self-inquiry exercises to inspire your mind to open to what is really going on inside. It's up to you to continue to use these tools and build upon them in order to experience continued success in your physical, emotional and spiritual health.

Now that you have discovered some of the foods that affect your body in a toxic way and/or create inflammation; continue to remove those foods from your daily routine. Keep your food journal handy so you can continue to document how you feel when you eat. Continue to talk to your body. Ask your body daily; what do you need from me? As you continue to change your diet; it may now be time to partner with your physician or chosen healer and begin to look at food allergies, or dietary needs that work with your body and specific blood type. And last but most important; pay attention to your emotions! Your emotional state is the unlock to most of your physical ailments. By being in tune with your emotions and working through them; even expressing them, you will find your physical well-being stays in balance and it is easier to manage your day to day routines.

Become aware – Come out of Samsara. Be willing to complete self-inquiry exercises. Practice mindfulness.

Become wise – Find the teachers, doctors and healers that you trust that can help you to begin your journey. Find out as much information as you can about your body and yourself. Learn all you can. Study different spiritual practices and find what works for you. Take different exercise courses to find what works for you. Read and Study.

Practice – You must practice all that you are learning. Meditating and practicing mindfulness daily. The more you practice the more solid you become in your Self and your Spirit. The practice is The Path and The Way.

TRUST – Faith is the most important piece. You have to trust in yourself and in the Divine. You have to trust that you are always safe in the hands of Spirit. When you do not trust you must go back to the beginning with self-inquiry. What is it that I do not trust?

FOOD SENSITIVITY TRACKINGTEMPLATE

Foods I ate today:

List any physical reactions to food or symptoms that appeared during the day.

What emotional and/or outside triggers affected your food choices today?

What foods did you decide to eliminate from your diet based on how they affected your body?

Date:

How did I feel physically before and after I ate?

What did you learn about your eating habits today?

ENLIGHTENMENT PIE
PURIFY. ENERGIZE. HEAL.

बाधा:

FOOD SENSITIVITY TRACKING TEMPLATE

Foods I ate today:

List any physical reactions to food or symptoms that appeared during the day.

What emotional and/or outside triggers affected your food choices today?

What foods did you decide to eliminate from your die based on how they affected your body?

Date:

How did I feel physically before and after I ate?

What did you learn about your eating habits today?

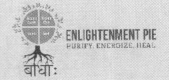

ENLIGHTENMENT PIE
PURIFY, ENERGIZE, HEAL

FOOD SENSITIVITY TRACKING TEMPLATE

Foods I ate today:

Date:

How did I feel physically before and after I ate?

List any physical reactions to food or symptoms that appeared during the day.

What emotional and/or outside triggers affected your food choices today?

What did you learn about your eating habits today?

What foods did you decide to eliminate from your die- based on how they affected your body?

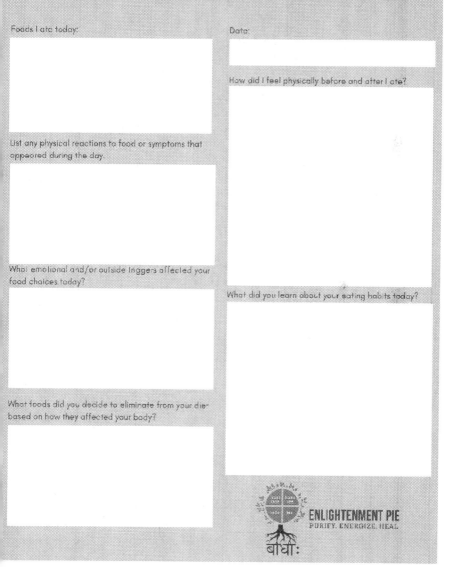

ENLIGHTENMENT PIE
PURIFY. ENERGIZE. HEAL.

FOOD SENSITIVITY TRACKING TEMPLATE

Foods I ate today:

Date:

List any physical reactions to food or symptoms that appeared during the day.

How did I feel physically before and after I ate?

What emotional and/or outside triggers affected your food choices today?

What did you learn about your eating habits today?

What foods did you decide to eliminate from your diet based on how they affected your body?

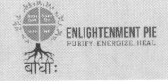

ENLIGHTENMENT PIE
PURIFY. ENERGIZE. HEAL.

बाधा:

FOOD SENSITIVITY TRACKING TEMPLATE

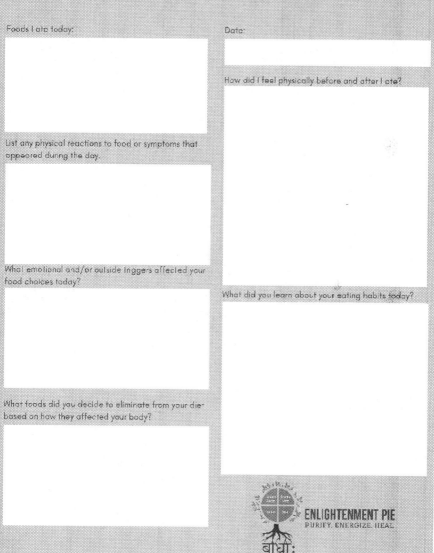

Foods I ate today:

Date:

List any physical reactions to food or symptoms that appeared during the day.

How did I feel physically before and after I ate?

What emotional and/or outside triggers affected your food choices today?

What did you learn about your eating habits today?

What foods did you decide to eliminate from your diet based on how they affected your body?

ENLIGHTENMENT PIE
PURIFY, ENERGIZE, HEAL

बाधा:

FOOD SENSITIVITY TRACKING TEMPLATE

Foods I ate today:

Date:

How did I feel physically before and after I ate?

List any physical reactions to food or symptoms that appeared during the day.

What emotional and/or outside triggers affected your food choices today?

What did you learn about your eating habits today?

What foods did you decide to eliminate from your diet based on how they affected your body?

ENLIGHTENMENT PIE
PURIFY. ENERGIZE. HEAL.

बाधा:

FOOD SENSITIVITY TRACKING TEMPLATE

Foods I ate today:

Date:

How did I feel physically before and after I ate?

List any physical reactions to food or symptoms that appeared during the day.

What emotional and/or outside triggers affected your food choices today?

What did you learn about your eating habits today?

What foods did you decide to eliminate from your diet based on how they affected your body?

ENLIGHTENMENT PIE
PURIFY. ENERGIZE. HEAL.

बाधा:

FOOD SENSITIVITY TRACKING TEMPLATE

Foods I ate today:

Date:

How did I feel physically before and after I ate?

List any physical reactions to food or symptoms that appeared during the day.

What emotional and/or outside triggers affected your food choices today?

What did you learn about your eating habits today?

What foods did you decide to eliminate from your diet based on how they affected your body?

ENLIGHTENMENT PIE
PURIFY. ENERGIZE. HEAL.

बाधा:

FOOD SENSITIVITY TRACKING TEMPLATE

Foods I ate today:

List any physical reactions to food or symptoms that appeared during the day.

What emotional and/or outside triggers affected your food choices today?

What foods did you decide to eliminate from your diet based on how they affected your body?

Date:

How did I feel physically before and after I ate?

What did you learn about your eating habits today?

ENLIGHTENMENT PIE
PURIFY. ENERGIZE. HEAL.

बाधा:

FOOD SENSITIVITY TRACKING TEMPLATE

Foods I ate today:

Date:

How did I feel physically before and after I ate?

List any physical reactions to food or symptoms that appeared during the day.

What emotional and/or outside triggers affected your food choices today?

What did you learn about your eating habits today?

What foods did you decide to eliminate from your diet based on how they affected your body?

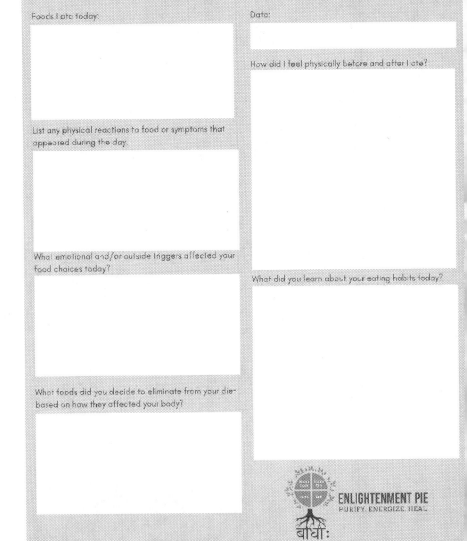

ENLIGHTENMENT PIE
PURIFY. ENERGIZE. HEAL.

बीधा:

FOOD SENSITIVITY TRACKING TEMPLATE

Foods I ate today:

Date:

How did I feel physically before and after I ate?

List any physical reactions to food or symptoms that appeared during the day.

What emotional and/or outside triggers affected your food choices today?

What did you learn about your eating habits today?

What foods did you decide to eliminate from your diet based on how they affected your body?

ENLIGHTENMENT PIE
PURIFY, ENERGIZE, HEAL

बाधा:

FOOD SENSITIVITY TRACKING TEMPLATE

Foods I ate today:

Date:

How did I feel physically before and after I ate?

List any physical reactions to food or symptoms that appeared during the day.

What emotional and/or outside triggers affected your food choices today?

What did you learn about your eating habits today?

What foods did you decide to eliminate from your diet based on how they affected your body?

ENLIGHTENMENT PIE
PURIFY. ENERGIZE. HEAL.

बाधा:

FOOD SENSITIVITY TRACKING TEMPLATE

Foods I ate today:

Date:

How did I feel physically before and after I ate?

List any physical reactions to food or symptoms that appeared during the day.

What emotional and/or outside triggers affected your food choices today?

What did you learn about your eating habits today?

What foods did you decide to eliminate from your diet based on how they affected your body?

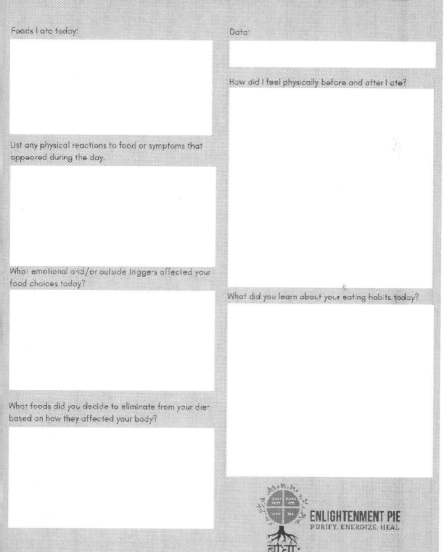

ENLIGHTENMENT PIE
PURIFY. ENERGIZE. HEAL.

बाधा:

FOOD SENSITIVITY TRACKING TEMPLATE

Foods I ate today:

Date:

How did I feel physically before and after I ate?

List any physical reactions to food or symptoms that appeared during the day.

What emotional and/or outside triggers affected your food choices today?

What did you learn about your eating habits today?

What foods did you decide to eliminate from your diet based on how they affected your body?

ENLIGHTENMENT PIE
PURIFY. ENERGIZE. HEAL

बाधाः

FOOD SENSITIVITY TRACKING TEMPLATE

Foods I ate today:

Date:

How did I feel physically before and after I ate?

List any physical reactions to food or symptoms that appeared during the day.

What emotional and/or outside triggers affected your food choices today?

What did you learn about your eating habits today?

What foods did you decide to eliminate from your diet based on how they affected your body?

ENLIGHTENMENT PIE
PURIFY. ENERGIZE. HEAL.

बाधा:

FOOD SENSITIVITY TRACKING TEMPLATE

Foods I ate today:

List any physical reactions to food or symptoms that appeared during the day.

What emotional and/or outside triggers affected your food choices today?

What foods did you decide to eliminate from your diet based on how they affected your body?

Date:

How did I feel physically before and after I ate?

What did you learn about your eating habits today?

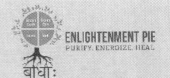

ENLIGHTENMENT PIE
PURIFY. ENERGIZE. HEAL.

बोधि:

FOOD SENSITIVITY TRACKING TEMPLATE

Foods I ate today:

Date:

List any physical reactions to food or symptoms that appeared during the day.

How did I feel physically before and after I ate?

What emotional and/or outside triggers affected your food choices today?

What did you learn about your eating habits today?

What foods did you decide to eliminate from your diet based on how they affected your body?

ENLIGHTENMENT PIE
PURIFY. ENERGIZE. HEAL

बाधाः

FOOD SENSITIVITY TRACKING TEMPLATE

Foods I ate today:

List any physical reactions to food or symptoms that appeared during the day.

What emotional and/or outside triggers affected your food choices today?

What foods did you decide to eliminate from your die- based on how they affected your body?

Date:

How did I feel physically before and after I ate?

What did you learn about your eating habits today?

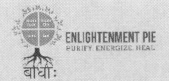

FOOD SENSITIVITY TRACKING TEMPLATE

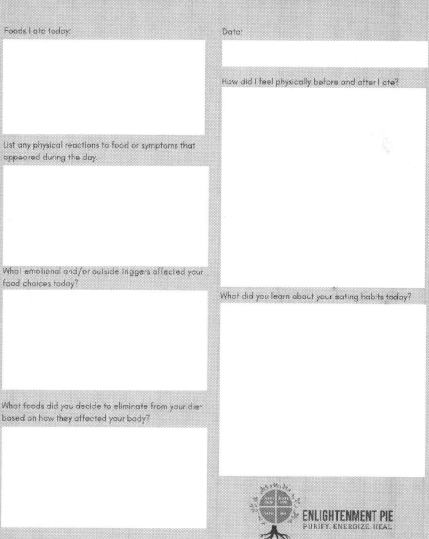

Foods I ate today:

Date:

How did I feel physically before and after I ate?

List any physical reactions to food or symptoms that appeared during the day.

What emotional and/or outside triggers affected your food choices today?

What did you learn about your eating habits today?

What foods did you decide to eliminate from your diet based on how they affected your body?

ENLIGHTENMENT PIE
PURIFY, ENERGIZE, HEAL

बाधा:

FOOD SENSITIVITY TRACKING TEMPLATE

Foods I ate today:

List any physical reactions to food or symptoms that appeared during the day.

What emotional and/or outside triggers affected your food choices today?

What foods did you decide to eliminate from your diet based on how they affected your body?

Date:

How did I feel physically before and after I ate?

What did you learn about your eating habits today?

ENLIGHTENMENT PIE
PURIFY. ENERGIZE. HEAL.

बाधा:

FOOD SENSITIVITY TRACKING TEMPLATE

Foods I ate today:

Date:

How did I feel physically before and after I ate?

List any physical reactions to food or symptoms that appeared during the day.

What emotional and/or outside triggers affected your food choices today?

What did you learn about your eating habits today?

What foods did you decide to eliminate from your diet based on how they affected your body?

ENLIGHTENMENT PIE
PURIFY. ENERGIZE. HEAL.

बाधा:

FOOD SENSITIVITY TRACKING TEMPLATE

Foods I ate today:

Date:

How did I feel physically before and after I ate?

List any physical reactions to food or symptoms that appeared during the day.

What emotional and/or outside triggers affected your food choices today?

What did you learn about your eating habits today?

What foods did you decide to eliminate from your diet based on how they affected your body?

ENLIGHTENMENT PIE
PURIFY. ENERGIZE. HEAL.

बाधा:

FOOD SENSITIVITY TRACKING TEMPLATE

Foods I ate today:

List any physical reactions to food or symptoms that appeared during the day.

What emotional and/or outside triggers affected your food choices today?

What foods did you decide to eliminate from your diet based on how they affected your body?

Date:

How did I feel physically before and after I ate?

What did you learn about your eating habits today?

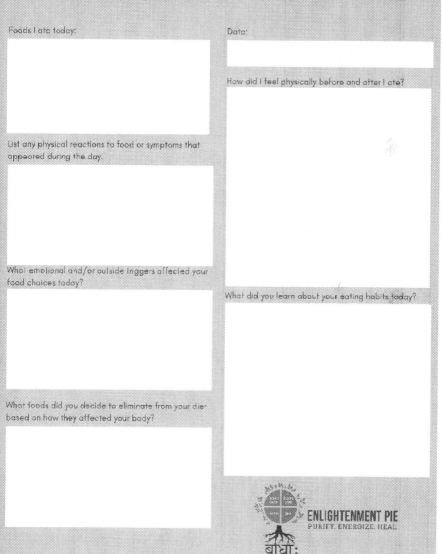

ENLIGHTENMENT PIE
PURIFY. ENERGIZE. HEAL.

बाधा:

FOOD SENSITIVITY TRACKING TEMPLATE

Foods I ate today:

Date:

How did I feel physically before and after I ate?

List any physical reactions to food or symptoms that appeared during the day.

What emotional and/or outside triggers affected your food choices today?

What did you learn about your eating habits today?

What foods did you decide to eliminate from your diet based on how they affected your body?

ENLIGHTENMENT PIE
PURIFY. ENERGIZE. HEAL

बाधा:

FOOD SENSITIVITY TRACKING TEMPLATE

Foods I ate today:

List any physical reactions to food or symptoms that appeared during the day.

What emotional and/or outside triggers affected your food choices today?

What foods did you decide to eliminate from your diet based on how they affected your body?

Date:

How did I feel physically before and after I ate?

What did you learn about your eating habits today?

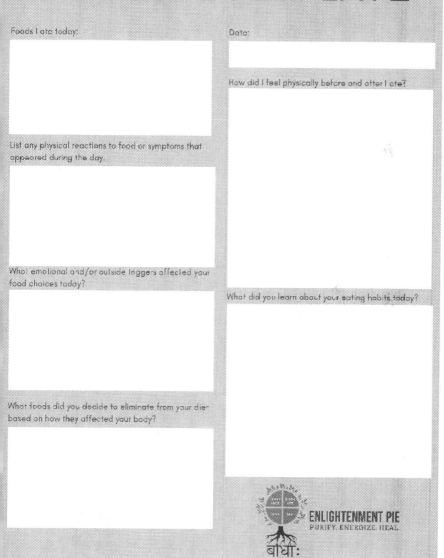

ENLIGHTENMENT PIE
PURIFY. ENERGIZE. HEAL.

बाधा:

FOOD SENSITIVITY TRACKING TEMPLATE

Foods I ate today:

List any physical reactions to food or symptoms that appeared during the day.

What emotional and/or outside triggers affected your food choices today?

What foods did you decide to eliminate from your diet based on how they affected your body?

Date:

How did I feel physically before and after I ate?

What did you learn about your eating habits today?

ENLIGHTENMENT PIE
PURIFY, ENERGIZE, HEAL

बाधा:

FOOD SENSITIVITY TRACKING TEMPLATE

Foods I ate today:

List any physical reactions to food or symptoms that appeared during the day.

What emotional and/or outside triggers affected your food choices today?

What foods did you decide to eliminate from your die- based on how they affected your body?

Date:

How did I feel physically before and after I ate?

What did you learn about your eating habits today?

ENLIGHTENMENT PIE
PURIFY. ENERGIZE. HEAL.

बाधा:

FOOD SENSITIVITY
TRACKING TEMPLATE

Foods I ate today:

Date:

How did I feel physically before and after I ate?

List any physical reactions to food or symptoms that appeared during the day.

What emotional and/or outside triggers affected your food choices today?

What did you learn about your eating habits today?

What foods did you decide to eliminate from your diet based on how they affected your body?

ENLIGHTENMENT PIE
PURIFY. ENERGIZE. HEAL.

बोधि:

FOOD SENSITIVITY TRACKING TEMPLATE

Foods I ate today:

List any physical reactions to food or symptoms that appeared during the day.

What emotional and/or outside triggers affected your food choices today?

What foods did you decide to eliminate from your die- based on how they affected your body?

Date:

How did I feel physically before and after I ate?

What did you learn about your eating habits today?

ENLIGHTENMENT PIE
PURIFY. ENERGIZE. HEAL

बाधाः

FOOD SENSITIVITY TRACKINGTEMPLATE

Foods I ate today:

Date:

How did I feel physically before and after I ate?

List any physical reactions to food or symptoms that appeared during the day.

What emotional and/or outside triggers affected your food choices today?

What did you learn about your eating habits today?

What foods did you decide to eliminate from your diet based on how they affected your body?

ENLIGHTENMENT PIE
PURIFY. ENERGIZE. HEAL.

बाधा:

FOOD SENSITIVITY TRACKING TEMPLATE

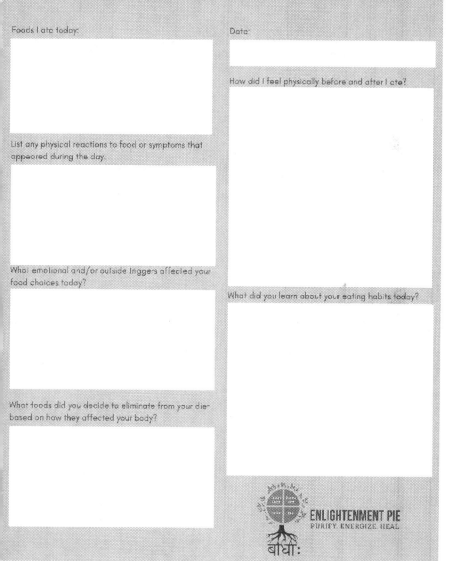

Foods I ate today:

Date:

List any physical reactions to food or symptoms that appeared during the day.

How did I feel physically before and after I ate?

What emotional and/or outside triggers affected your food choices today?

What did you learn about your eating habits today?

What foods did you decide to eliminate from your diet based on how they affected your body?

ENLIGHTENMENT PIE
PURIFY. ENERGIZE. HEAL.

बाधाः

FOOD SENSITIVITY TRACKING TEMPLATE

Foods I ate today:

Date:

How did I feel physically before and after I ate?

List any physical reactions to food or symptoms that appeared during the day.

What emotional and/or outside triggers affected your food choices today?

What did you learn about your eating habits today?

What foods did you decide to eliminate from your diet based on how they affected your body?

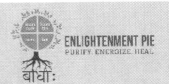

ENLIGHTENMENT PIE
PURIFY. ENERGIZE. HEAL.

बाधाः

FOOD SENSITIVITY TRACKING TEMPLATE

Foods I ate today:

List any physical reactions to food or symptoms that appeared during the day.

What emotional and/or outside triggers affected your food choices today?

What foods did you decide to eliminate from your diet based on how they affected your body?

Date:

How did I feel physically before and after I ate?

What did you learn about your eating habits today?

ENLIGHTENMENT PIE
PURIFY. ENERGIZE. HEAL

बाधा:

FOOD SENSITIVITY TRACKING TEMPLATE

Foods I ate today:

Date:

How did I feel physically before and after I ate?

List any physical reactions to food or symptoms that appeared during the day.

What emotional and/or outside triggers affected your food choices today?

What did you learn about your eating habits today?

What foods did you decide to eliminate from your diet based on how they affected your body?

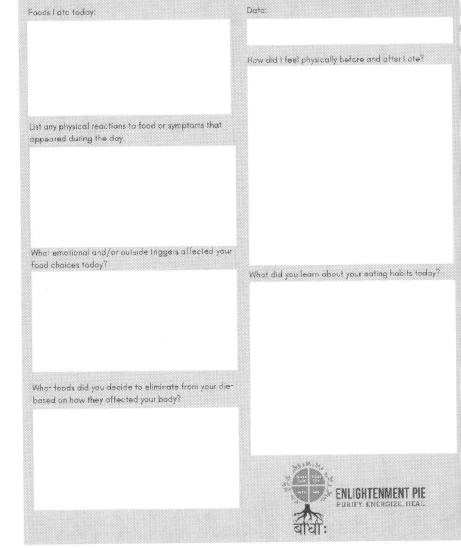

ENLIGHTENMENT PIE
PURIFY. ENERGIZE. HEAL

बाधा:

FOOD SENSITIVITY TRACKING TEMPLATE

Foods I ate today:

List any physical reactions to food or symptoms that appeared during the day.

What emotional and/or outside triggers affected your food choices today?

What foods did you decide to eliminate from your diet based on how they affected your body?

Date:

How did I feel physically before and after I ate?

What did you learn about your eating habits today?

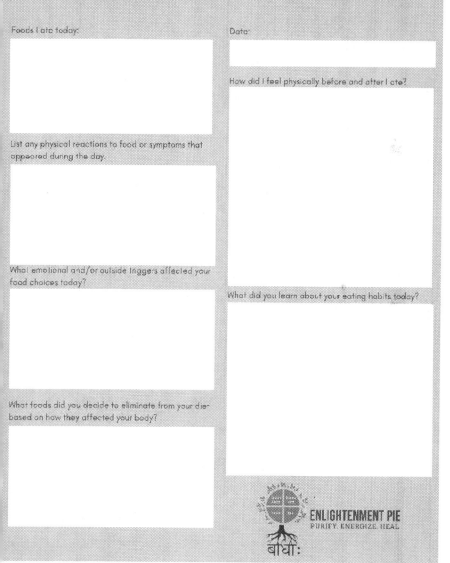

ENLIGHTENMENT PIE
PURIFY. ENERGIZE. HEAL

FOOD SENSITIVITY TRACKING TEMPLATE

Foods I ate today:

Date:

How did I feel physically before and after I ate?

List any physical reactions to food or symptoms that appeared during the day.

What emotional and/or outside triggers affected your food choices today?

What did you learn about your eating habits today?

What foods did you decide to eliminate from your diet based on how they affected your body?

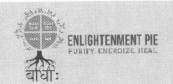

ENLIGHTENMENT PIE
PURIFY. ENERGIZE. HEAL.

बोधि:

FOOD SENSITIVITY TRACKINGTEMPLATE

Foods I ate today:

List any physical reactions to food or symptoms that appeared during the day.

What emotional and/or outside triggers affected your food choices today?

What foods did you decide to eliminate from your die-based on how they affected your body?

Date:

How did I feel physically before and after I ate?

What did you learn about your eating habits today?

ENLIGHTENMENT PIE
PURIFY. ENERGIZE. HEAL.

बोधा:

FOOD SENSITIVITY TRACKING TEMPLATE

Foods I ate today:

Date:

How did I feel physically before and after I ate?

List any physical reactions to food or symptoms that appeared during the day.

What emotional and/or outside triggers affected your food choices today?

What did you learn about your eating habits today?

What foods did you decide to eliminate from your diet based on how they affected your body?

ENLIGHTENMENT PIE
PURIFY. ENERGIZE. HEAL.

बाधाः

FOOD SENSITIVITY TRACKING TEMPLATE

Foods I ate today:

Date:

How did I feel physically before and after I ate?

List any physical reactions to food or symptoms that appeared during the day.

What emotional and/or outside triggers affected your food choices today?

What did you learn about your eating habits today?

What foods did you decide to eliminate from your diet based on how they affected your body?

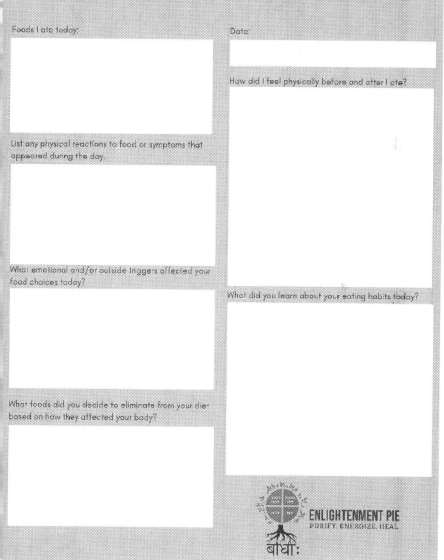

ENLIGHTENMENT PIE
PURIFY. ENERGIZE. HEAL.
बाधा:

FOOD SENSITIVITY TRACKING TEMPLATE

Foods I ate today:

Date:

How did I feel physically before and after I ate?

List any physical reactions to food or symptoms that appeared during the day.

What emotional and/or outside triggers affected your food choices today?

What did you learn about your eating habits today?

What foods did you decide to eliminate from your diet based on how they affected your body?

ENLIGHTENMENT PIE
PURIFY, ENERGIZE, HEAL

बाधा:

FOOD SENSITIVITY TRACKING TEMPLATE

Foods I ate today:

Date:

How did I feel physically before and after I ate?

List any physical reactions to food or symptoms that appeared during the day.

What emotional and/or outside triggers affected your food choices today?

What did you learn about your eating habits today?

What foods did you decide to eliminate from your diet based on how they affected your body?

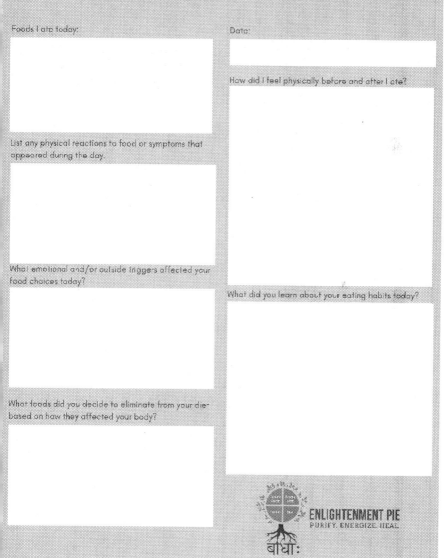

ENLIGHTENMENT PIE
PURIFY. ENERGIZE. HEAL

बाधा:

FOOD SENSITIVITY TRACKING TEMPLATE

Foods I ate today:

Date:

How did I feel physically before and after I ate?

List any physical reactions to food or symptoms that appeared during the day.

What emotional and/or outside triggers affected your food choices today?

What did you learn about your eating habits today?

What foods did you decide to eliminate from your diet based on how they affected your body?

ENLIGHTENMENT PIE
PURIFY, ENERGIZE, HEAL

बाधा:

FOOD SENSITIVITY TRACKING TEMPLATE

Foods I ate today:

List any physical reactions to food or symptoms that appeared during the day.

What emotional and/or outside triggers affected your food choices today?

What foods did you decide to eliminate from your diet based on how they affected your body?

Date:

How did I feel physically before and after I ate?

What did you learn about your eating habits today?

ENLIGHTENMENT PIE
PURIFY. ENERGIZE. HEAL

बाधाः

FOOD SENSITIVITY TRACKING TEMPLATE

Foods I ate today:

Date:

How did I feel physically before and after I ate?

List any physical reactions to food or symptoms that appeared during the day.

What emotional and/or outside triggers affected your food choices today?

What did you learn about your eating habits today?

What foods did you decide to eliminate from your diet based on how they affected your body?

ENLIGHTENMENT PIE
PURIFY. ENERGIZE. HEAL.

बाधा:

FOOD SENSITIVITY TRACKING TEMPLATE

Foods I ate today:

Date:

How did I feel physically before and after I ate?

List any physical reactions to food or symptoms that appeared during the day.

What emotional and/or outside triggers affected your food choices today?

What did you learn about your eating habits today?

What foods did you decide to eliminate from your diet based on how they affected your body?

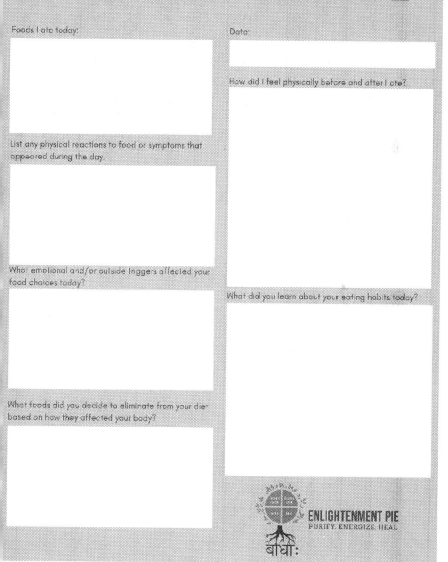

ENLIGHTENMENT PIE
PURIFY. ENERGIZE. HEAL

बाधा:

About the Author

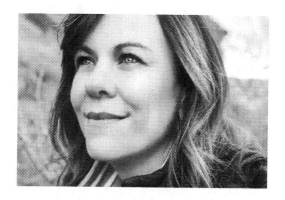

Toxicity is surfacing at an ever-increasing rate to be purified and released so global consciousness can continue to expand. On a personal level, we also are being called to purify our bodies and minds to reach new levels of awareness. Over the past decade I have been blessed to work with many different clients, including my own personal journey, to remove toxic energies from our lives and fine tune our vibration. For me the result has been a physical loss of over 100 pounds and a completely new direction in work and relationships.

Spiritual and psychic gifts came to me through the generations of women in my family. I am the fourth generation of an incredible group of gifted healers, mediums and channels. I am able to give guidance to help heal your life through psychic readings, visiting the Akashic Records, connecting to teachers and loved ones and journeying to different Lokas or dimensions specialize in helping you transition out of or recover from toxic situations such as; toxic work environments, home environments, toxic relationships and food sensitivities and toxicities. We will work together to identify the spiritual and emotional cause of attraction of these negative situations and begin to heal them through soul retrieval, self-inquiry and spiritual practices.

I have a personal relationship with mold toxins and fungus. Their metaphysical reason to exist in a body is holding on to your past and allowing toxic energies to feed on your energy. For me, this was a direct correlation to the toxic relationships I had built and my own food addiction and patterns of codependency. I have found there are many sensitives managing these same issues. I have a special program for those of you suffering from mold and fungus dysfunction. This involves detox support for your physical body as well as emotional support as you move through the detox. The most important piece is using self-inquiry to identify the areas in your childhood that may have created these patterns; such as childhood abuse or addictive behaviors in your family. Once these areas are identified we are able to journey back to those ages and complete soul retrieval to begin to bring these fragments back to your Self to become whole.

It is my passion to cultivate compassion and loving kindness and it is through my Faith in the teachers and Gurus that I have been able to be healed. I now offer service to you, so we can all live in balance, health and vitality and increase conscious awareness for the greater good of all sentient beings.

Lisa has an Associates of Applied Science Degree in Culinary Arts from the Art Institute of Colorado and is certified in Nutritional Cooking by the American Culinary Federation; Recognized by the National Association of Psychics and Mediums, Ordained Minister through the Universal Life Church and is a Certified Professional Tarot Reader through the Tarot Certification Board of America. Lisa also completed the Berkeley Psychic Institute's Program through Psychic Horizons in Boulder, CO.